Trauma-Focused CBT for Girls

A Comprehensive Guide to Healing Trauma in Girl Child

Sophie Conner

A Comprehensive Guide to Healing Trauma in Girl Child

Sophie Conner

Copyright © (2023) Sophie Conner. All rights reserved.

No part of this book may be reproduced, stored in a retrieval system, or transmitted in any form or by any means, electronic, mechanical, photocopying, recording, or otherwise, without prior written permission of the publisher, except for the inclusion of brief quotations in a review.

Published by: **True Pen Publisher**
4700 HIGHWAY 280 EAST SUITE 5
BIRMINGHAM, SHELBY, AL 35244
UNITED STATES

Cover design by Jenson Brooks
Printed in the United States of America

For more information, visit www.risepublisher.com

DEDICATION

To all the resilient girls and women who have endured trauma, you are stronger than you know. May this book be a beacon of hope and healing on your journey towards reclaiming your power and rebuilding your life. Your courage inspires me, and it is my honor to contribute to your path of recovery and transformation.

With deepest admiration and respect,

Sophie Conner

Contents

Title page ii
Copyright page ii
DEDICATION iv
PREFACE vii
Understanding Trauma and Its Impact on Girls 1

Part I 7
Foundations of Trauma-Focused CBT: 7
Trauma-Informed Care 13
Assessment and Treatment Planning 17

Part II 23
Therapeutic Techniques for Trauma: 23
Psychoeducation and Skills Building 23
Trauma Processing and Cognitive Restructuring 28
Behavioral Activation and Experiential Techniques ... 32
Addressing Common Trauma Responses 37

Part III 43
Working with Specific Populations: 43
Trauma in Childhood and Adolescence 43
Intersectionality and Cultural Competence 49
Trauma in High-Risk Populations 54

Part IV..61
Clinical Applications and Special Considerations.......61
Integrating Trauma-Focused CBT with Other
Therapies...61
Working with Caregivers and Support Systems...........67
Ethical and Legal Considerations 73

Conclusion...81

PREFACE

Trauma knows no bounds and can affect anyone, regardless of age, gender, or background. However, the impact of trauma on girls and women is unique and often goes unrecognized or misunderstood. As a therapist specializing in cognitive-behavioral therapy (CBT), I have witnessed firsthand the transformative power of trauma-focused CBT in helping girls and young women heal from the depths of their traumatic experiences.

In my practice, I have worked with countless individuals who have endured trauma in its many forms—from childhood abuse and neglect to community violence and natural disasters. Through their courage and resilience, they have shown me the profound potential for healing and growth that lies within each person. It is this hope and resilience that I aim to capture and share through this book.

"Trauma-Focused CBT for Girls" is a comprehensive guide designed to empower therapists, counselors, and mental health professionals working with trauma-exposed girls. By providing a deep understanding of the intersection between trauma and female development, this book offers practical tools and strategies rooted in trauma-focused CBT. My goal is to bridge the gap between theory and practice, offering a roadmap for therapists to navigate the complex journey of trauma recovery alongside their young clients.

Within these pages, readers will find a wealth of information, from the foundational principles of CBT and trauma-informed care to specific therapeutic techniques and interventions. I have also included real-world case examples and personal reflections to illustrate the application of these concepts in clinical practice. Additionally, special attention is given to working with diverse populations, recognizing the importance of cultural competence in trauma-informed therapy.

It is my sincere hope that this book will not only enhance the therapeutic skills of professionals but also contribute to a broader understanding of trauma and its impact on girls and women. Together, we can create a world where trauma is recognized, addressed, and healed, empowering individuals to reclaim their lives and reach their full potential.

I invite you to embark on this journey with me as we explore the transformative power of trauma-focused CBT and work towards a brighter future for trauma survivors.

Sophie Conner

Understanding Trauma and Its Impact on Girls

Trauma is an intricate and multifaceted concept that has captured the attention of mental health professionals, researchers, and society at large. It is a profound and often life-altering experience that can leave deep imprints on an individual's psyche and overall well-being. In this book, we will delve into the complex world of trauma, exploring its definition, prevalence, and the unique ways it affects girls and women. By shedding light on the psychological and physiological consequences of trauma, we aim to foster a deeper understanding of the challenges faced by trauma survivors and the pathways to healing. So, let's embark on this journey together as we unravel the complexities of trauma and its impact on girls, paving the way for empathy, support, and effective intervention.

Trauma can be understood as an emotional response to a deeply distressing or disturbing event or series of events that pose a threat to an individual's physical, emotional, or psychological well-being. It encompasses a wide range of experiences, from natural disasters and accidents to abuse, violence, and loss. At its core, trauma involves a sense of overwhelming stress and a feeling of powerlessness or loss of control.

The impact of trauma is not limited to a single incident but can extend far beyond, influencing an individual's thoughts, emotions, behaviors, and relationships. It is crucial to recognize that trauma is subjective, and what may be traumatic for one person might not be for another. This subjectivity arises from variations in personal backgrounds, cultural contexts, resilience, and available support systems. Thus, a comprehensive understanding of trauma requires a nuanced and individualized perspective.

Trauma knows no boundaries and can affect anyone, regardless of age, race, or social status. However, research and statistical analyses reveal a concerning prevalence of trauma among girls and women. According to the National Child Traumatic Stress Network, an estimated 61% of boys and 51% of girls in the United States have experienced at least one traumatic event by the age of 16. These events can include accidents, natural disasters, community violence, or personal losses.

While these statistics are already significant, they only scratch the surface. The true extent of trauma exposure among girls and women is likely even higher due to underreporting and the hidden nature of certain traumatic experiences, such as sexual abuse or domestic violence. Studies indicate that girls and women are at a higher risk of experiencing certain types of trauma, particularly those involving interpersonal violence and sexual assault. This heightened vulnerability underscores the urgent need for trauma-informed approaches and interventions specifically tailored to meet the unique needs of this population.

The impact of trauma on girls can manifest in various psychological ways, often presenting as a complex interplay of emotions, thoughts, and behaviors. Girls who have experienced trauma may struggle with anxiety, depression, post-traumatic stress disorder (PTSD), or other trauma-related disorders. They might exhibit symptoms such as intrusive memories or flashbacks, avoidance of trauma-related triggers, negative changes in cognition and mood, and heightened arousal or reactivity.

Trauma can also disrupt a girl's sense of self and impact her ability to regulate emotions effectively. She may develop negative core beliefs about herself, others, and the world, leading to low self-esteem, self-blame, or a sense of worthlessness. Trauma can disrupt healthy attachment patterns, affecting her relationships with peers, family, and authority figures. Additionally, trauma can contribute to difficulties in school, impaired social functioning, and an increased risk of engaging in risky behaviors.

The impact of trauma extends beyond the psychological realm, as it also has significant physiological consequences, particularly during critical periods of female development. Adverse childhood experiences (ACEs), which include various forms of trauma, have been linked to what is known as toxic stress.

This prolonged activation of the stress response system can have long-lasting effects on brain development, immune function, and even epigenetic changes.

When girls experience trauma, their stress response systems can become dysregulated, leading to heightened reactivity and difficulties with emotional and behavioral self-regulation. They may exhibit increased levels of the stress hormone cortisol, which, over time, can impact their overall health and contribute to physical ailments such as digestive issues, headaches, or sleep disturbances. Trauma can also disrupt healthy hormonal balance, affecting reproductive health and increasing the risk of gynecological problems.

The impact of trauma on the developing brain is particularly noteworthy. Trauma can influence the architecture and functioning of key regions involved in emotional processing, decision-making, and impulse control. This can lead to challenges with executive functioning, attention, and memory. Additionally, trauma can shape the development of neural pathways involved in social and emotional learning, potentially impacting a girl's ability to form secure attachments and navigate social relationships effectively.

Girls facing trauma often encounter unique challenges and barriers to healing. They may internalize their emotions and suffer in silence due to societal expectations of femininity and the pressure to appear "perfect." Shame and self-blame are common responses, especially in cases of sexual abuse or assault, which can hinder their ability to seek help or disclose their experiences.

Gender stereotypes and biases can further complicate the trauma recovery process for girls. They may face additional layers of stigma, blame, or disbelief, especially in cultures that emphasize female passivity or dismiss female experiences. These societal factors can create a sense of isolation and hinder their access to supportive resources and effective treatment.

Despite the profound impact of trauma, it is important to recognize that healing is possible. Girls possess inherent resilience, and with the right support, they can navigate the path toward recovery and post-traumatic growth. Trauma-informed approaches, such as trauma-focused cognitive-behavioral therapy (TF-CBT), are designed to empower survivors, helping them process their experiences, challenge negative cognitions, and develop adaptive coping strategies.

By raising awareness, educating ourselves, and advocating for trauma-informed practices, we can create a supportive environment that fosters resilience and healing. This includes addressing the root causes of trauma, promoting gender equality, and ensuring access to specialized mental health services for girls and women. Together, we can work towards breaking the cycle of trauma and empowering survivors to reclaim their lives with strength and hope.

Trauma is a complex and far-reaching phenomenon that leaves indelible marks on the lives of girls and women. By recognizing the prevalence and unique impact of trauma on female development, we take a crucial step towards fostering empathy, understanding, and effective intervention. As we shine a light on the psychological and physiological consequences of trauma, we also acknowledge the resilience and strength inherent in survivors.

Healing is a journey, and with the right support, girls can navigate the path from trauma to recovery. This section sets the foundation for a deeper exploration of trauma-focused cognitive-behavioral therapy and its potential to facilitate healing and transformation. As we continue this exploration, let us remain mindful of the unique needs of girls, advocating for trauma-informed practices that honor their resilience and empower them to rewrite their narratives with courage and hope.

Part I

Foundations of Trauma-Focused CBT:

Welcome to the captivating world of Cognitive-Behavioral Therapy, a therapeutic approach that has transformed the lives of countless individuals struggling with a myriad of mental health challenges. CBT is like a lighthouse shining a guiding light through the fog of confusion and distress, offering hope and a path forward toward healing. In the following pages, we will delve into the core principles of CBT, understanding how it works and why it has become one of the most widely recognized and effective therapeutic modalities. So, buckle up as we embark on this enlightening journey together!

At its core, Cognitive-Behavioral Therapy is grounded in the belief that our thoughts, feelings, and behaviors are intricately interconnected. This insight forms the foundation of the cognitive model, which proposes that our perceptions and interpretations of events significantly influence our emotional and behavioral responses. In simpler terms, the way we think about things can impact how we feel and act.

For example, imagine you're a teenager facing an important exam. If you think, "I always fail math tests; I'm just not good at it," your resulting feelings might be anxiety and discouragement. This emotional state could then lead to behaviors such as avoiding study sessions or procrastinating instead of seeking help. CBT aims to help individuals recognize and challenge these unhelpful thought patterns, offering a more balanced perspective that can lead to improved emotional well-being and effective problem-solving behaviors.

The Therapeutic Trio: Thoughts, Feelings, and Actions

One of the most powerful concepts in CBT is the recognition that our thoughts, feelings, and actions are all part of a dynamic system. When one element is affected, it creates a ripple effect on the others. Let's break it down:

- **Thoughts:** These are the beliefs, interpretations, and perceptions we have about ourselves, others, and the world around us. Thoughts can be conscious or unconscious, and they influence how we process and react to our experiences. In CBT, we explore and challenge unhelpful or distorted thinking patterns, often referred to as cognitive distortions. Examples include all-or-nothing thinking ("I never do anything right"), catastrophizing ("This tiny mistake will ruin everything"), or mind reading ("My friends think I'm boring").

- **Feelings**: Our emotions are the result of our thoughts and experiences. They provide valuable information about our inner world and can range from joy and excitement to sadness and anger. In CBT, we acknowledge and validate these emotions while also helping individuals develop healthy coping strategies. The goal is not to eliminate negative emotions but to manage and respond to them effectively.

- **Actions**: Our behaviors, or actions, are the observable responses to our thoughts and feelings. They can be adaptive, helping us achieve our goals, or maladaptive, perpetuating a cycle of distress. CBT focuses on behavior change by encouraging individuals to experiment with new, more constructive actions that align with their values and goals.

The CBT Toolbox: Techniques and Strategies

The beauty of CBT lies in its practical and actionable techniques. Think of it as a therapist's toolbox filled with an array of tools designed to address specific challenges. Here's a glimpse into some of the most commonly used techniques:

- **Cognitive Restructuring:** This involves identifying and challenging unhelpful thoughts. Therapists guide clients in recognizing cognitive distortions and replacing them with more balanced and realistic thoughts. It's like fine-tuning the lens through which we view the world.

- **Behavioral Activation:** Here, the focus is on increasing engagement in values-driven behaviors. Clients are encouraged to take small, gradual steps toward activities that bring a sense of fulfillment and purpose. This might include scheduling enjoyable activities, setting achievable goals, or challenging avoidance behaviors.

- **Exposure Therapy:** This technique is particularly powerful in treating anxiety disorders and trauma. It involves gradual exposure to feared stimuli or memories in a safe and controlled manner, helping individuals confront their fears and build resilience.

- **Relaxation and Mindfulness Techniques:** Teaching clients relaxation strategies, such as deep breathing, progressive muscle relaxation, or mindfulness practices, equips them with tools to manage stress and emotional overwhelm. These techniques often complement other CBT interventions.

The therapeutic relationship in CBT is a unique and collaborative partnership. Therapists create a safe, non-judgmental space where clients feel empowered to explore their thoughts and emotions. Unlike traditional psychoanalytic approaches, CBT emphasizes a more active and directive role for the therapist, often involving homework assignments and in-session exercises.

In this collaborative journey, therapists act as guides, educators, and supporters. They provide structure and guidance while encouraging clients to take an active role in their healing process. The relationship is based on mutual respect, openness, and a shared commitment to achieving the client's goals.

One of the hallmarks of CBT is its flexibility and adaptability. While the core principles remain consistent, therapists tailor the approach to meet the unique needs of each client. This might involve integrating elements from other therapeutic modalities or adapting techniques for specific populations, such as children, adolescents, or individuals with co-occurring disorders.

CBT is a highly individualized process, recognizing that each person brings their own set of experiences, strengths, and challenges. Therapists work collaboratively with clients to set personalized goals, ensuring that the treatment plan aligns with their values and desired outcomes.

CBT has earned its reputation as an evidence-based practice, backed by decades of scientific research. Numerous studies have demonstrated the effectiveness of CBT in treating a wide range of mental health concerns, including depression, anxiety disorders, trauma-related conditions, and substance use disorders. The therapeutic techniques employed in CBT have been rigorously tested and refined, ensuring their efficacy and applicability across diverse populations.

The ongoing research and development in CBT ensure that therapists can offer their clients the most up-to-date and effective interventions. This evidence-based foundation provides a solid ground for therapists and clients alike, fostering confidence in the therapeutic process and expected outcomes.

While CBT has proven highly effective, it's important to acknowledge its limitations. CBT may not be the best fit for every individual or every concern. For example, it may be less effective for individuals with severe psychosis or those primarily seeking insight and self-exploration rather than structured techniques. Additionally, the success of CBT relies on the client's willingness to engage in the process actively, including completing homework assignments and practicing new skills between sessions.

Furthermore, cultural considerations play a crucial role in the application of CBT. Therapists must be mindful of cultural differences in expression, communication styles, and conceptualizations of mental health. Adapting CBT to honor and incorporate cultural contexts is essential for its successful implementation across diverse populations.

Cognitive-Behavioral Therapy is a dynamic and versatile therapeutic approach that has changed the landscape of mental health treatment. By recognizing the interplay between thoughts, feelings, and actions, CBT empowers individuals to challenge unhelpful thinking patterns, develop healthier coping strategies, and lead more fulfilling lives.

As you continue on this therapeutic journey, whether as a therapist or an individual seeking healing, remember that CBT offers a beacon of hope and a path toward positive change. Embrace the principles and techniques shared in this section, and together, we can create a brighter future for those struggling with the weight of mental health challenges. Let CBT be the guiding light on the path toward healing and self-discovery!

Trauma-Informed Care

Trauma-informed care is a fundamental concept that underpins our approach to healing and forms the very foundation of this book. It's an essential paradigm shift in how we understand and respond to trauma, and it's about time we dive into this transformative perspective. So, let's explore what it truly means to provide trauma-informed care and how it can revolutionize the way we support girls on their journey of healing.

At its core, trauma-informed care is about recognizing the widespread impact of trauma and responding in a way that promotes healing, resilience, and empowerment. It's a holistic approach that acknowledges the deep and lasting effects trauma can have on an individual's emotional, physical, and psychological well-being. By adopting this lens, we can create safe, supportive, and responsive environments that facilitate recovery and growth.

Creating a safe space is paramount. For individuals who have experienced trauma, feeling secure and protected is often a significant challenge. Trauma can disrupt one's sense of safety and trust, making it difficult to form healthy attachments and connections. As therapists, we must be attuned to this and intentionally cultivate an environment that feels physically, emotionally, and psychologically safe. This means ensuring confidentiality, setting clear boundaries, and establishing predictability and consistency in our interactions. By doing so, we provide a sense of stability and security, allowing our clients to begin the process of healing without fear of judgment or re-traumatization.

Addressing power dynamics is another crucial aspect of trauma-informed care. Trauma often involves an abuse of power, leaving individuals feeling disempowered and vulnerable. In our therapeutic relationships, it's essential that we recognize and respect the inherent power imbalance that exists. We must actively work to minimize this power differential by fostering collaboration, choice, and autonomy. Encouraging open communication, seeking informed consent, and involving clients in decision-making processes are all ways to restore a sense of control and agency, which is often lost during traumatic experiences.

Empowerment is a key pillar of trauma-informed care. It's about helping individuals regain a sense of self-worth, strength, and the belief that they have the capacity to heal and thrive. We do this by recognizing and building upon their inherent resilience. Resilience is not about minimizing the impact of trauma but rather understanding that individuals possess inner resources and strengths that can be harnessed for healing. By identifying and nurturing these strengths, we empower our clients to become active participants in their recovery and agents of change in their lives.

Trauma-informed care also involves a deep understanding of the neurobiology of trauma and its impact on the brain and body. When individuals experience trauma, their stress response systems can become dysregulated, leading to a heightened state of arousal and reactivity. By incorporating trauma-sensitive practices, such as mindfulness, grounding techniques, and somatic awareness, we can help clients regulate their nervous systems and develop healthier coping strategies. This not only enhances their sense of safety and self-control but also improves their ability to engage in the therapeutic process more effectively.

Cultural humility plays a vital role in trauma-informed care. We must recognize that trauma intersects with various social identities, including race, ethnicity, gender, and sexual orientation. Cultural contexts and experiences shape how individuals express and cope with trauma. As therapists, it's imperative that we examine our own biases, privilege, and cultural competence. By embracing a culturally humble approach, we can create safe and inclusive spaces, adapt therapeutic techniques to meet diverse needs, and foster a sense of belonging for all.

Lastly, trauma-informed care extends beyond the individual and considers the broader systems and environments in which they exist. Trauma can impact families, communities, and societal structures. By adopting a systems perspective, we can advocate for social change, challenge systemic injustices, and promote trauma-informed practices in schools, healthcare settings, and beyond. This holistic view acknowledges the interconnectedness of trauma and encourages collaboration among professionals to support individuals in all aspects of their lives.

Trauma-informed care is a transformative approach that shifts our perspective and practice. It calls on us to create safe and empowering environments, address power dynamics, and promote resilience. By embracing these principles, we can facilitate healing, restore hope, and empower individuals to reclaim their lives after trauma. As you continue reading, remember that trauma-informed care is a guiding light on the path toward healing—a beacon that illuminates the way forward, fostering resilience and the potential for profound transformation.

Assessment and Treatment Planning

As a therapist embarking on the journey of trauma-focused cognitive-behavioral therapy (TF-CBT) with your young client, the initial assessment and treatment planning phase sets the stage for the entire therapeutic process. This crucial step provides a solid foundation for the work ahead and ensures that you truly understand the unique needs and experiences of the individual sitting across from you. So, let's dive into the intricate art of assessment and treatment planning, and I'll guide you through this essential aspect of TF- CBT step by step.

Understanding the Importance of Comprehensive Assessment

Think of the assessment phase as the foundation of a house. It needs to be solid, stable, and carefully constructed to support the entire structure. Similarly, a comprehensive trauma assessment provides the necessary insights and information to guide your treatment decisions and ensure they are tailored to your client's specific needs. It helps you understand the nature and extent of the trauma they have experienced, its impact on their thoughts, feelings, behaviors, and relationships, and any underlying vulnerabilities or strengths that may influence the therapeutic process.

Conducting the Trauma Assessment

When conducting a trauma assessment, it's important to create a safe, non-judgmental, and empathetic environment. Begin by gathering background information, including personal and family history, educational and medical background, and any previous mental health or substance use concerns. Explore the client's current life circumstances, supports, and stressors. Then, you can delve into the specifics of their trauma history.

Ask open-ended questions to encourage a detailed account of the traumatic event(s). It's important to assess for different types of trauma, such as acute trauma (e.g., accidents, natural disasters), chronic trauma (e.g., ongoing abuse, neglect), and complex trauma (resulting from repeated and prolonged traumatic experiences). Inquire about the client's reactions during and after the trauma, including any physical, emotional, cognitive, and behavioral responses. Understand the impact of the trauma on their daily functioning, relationships, and overall well-being.

Use validated assessment tools and screening measures to aid in your evaluation. These tools can help identify specific trauma-related disorders, such as post-traumatic stress disorder (PTSD), depression, or anxiety. They can also provide insights into the client's current symptoms, functioning, and areas of concern. Some commonly used assessments in TF-CBT include trauma-specific measures like the Trauma Symptoms Checklist for Children (TSCC) or the Child PTSD Symptom Scale, as well as general mental health screening tools like the Beck Depression Inventory or the Anxiety Disorders Interview Schedule for Children.

Developing a Comprehensive Case Formulation

Now, let's bring all the pieces of the puzzle together and develop a comprehensive case formulation. This involves integrating the information gathered during the assessment to create a coherent understanding of your client's presenting concerns, strengths, and treatment needs. A case formulation is more than just a list of symptoms or a diagnosis; it's a narrative that makes sense of the client's experiences and guides your treatment approach.

Consider the biological, psychological, social, and cultural factors that may contribute to your client's trauma responses and current functioning. Explore the interplay between the traumatic event(s) and their thoughts, feelings, and behaviors. For example, a young girl who has experienced sexual abuse may develop negative beliefs about herself, leading to low self-esteem, anxiety, and difficulties in relationships. Understand the maintaining factors that perpetuate their current struggles and identify potential protective factors that can support their healing journey.

Creating a Tailored Treatment Plan

The treatment plan is your roadmap for the therapeutic journey ahead. It outlines the specific goals, objectives, and interventions that will guide your work together. Collaboratively developing the treatment plan with your client and their caregivers (when appropriate) ensures a sense of shared understanding and investment in the process.

Begin by identifying the priority treatment goals. These goals should be specific, measurable, achievable, relevant, and time-bound (SMART goals). For example, a goal might be "Reduce the frequency and intensity of PTSD symptoms related to the traumatic event within the next three months." Then, break down the goal into smaller, measurable objectives. These objectives represent the steps needed to achieve the overall goal.

Select evidence-based interventions and techniques that align with TF-CBT and address the specific needs identified in the assessment and case formulation. For instance, if emotional regulation is a concern, you might incorporate mindfulness and relaxation techniques. If cognitive distortions are contributing to negative self-beliefs, you would incorporate cognitive restructuring strategies. Ensure that your treatment plan is flexible and adaptable, allowing for adjustments as your client's needs evolve throughout therapy.

Engaging Your Client and Caregivers

Involving your client and their caregivers in the treatment planning process is essential for fostering investment and motivation. Collaboratively set goals and discuss the rationale behind the chosen interventions. Provide psychoeducation about trauma and its effects, normalizing their experiences and empowering them with knowledge. When working with younger clients, it's crucial to use age-appropriate language and involve them in a developmentally appropriate manner.

For caregivers, provide education about trauma, its impact, and the role they can play in supporting their child's healing journey. Caregivers can be invaluable allies in the therapeutic process, and their involvement often enhances treatment outcomes. Address any concerns or misconceptions they may have and offer guidance on how they can best support their child both during and outside of therapy sessions.

The assessment and treatment planning phase is a critical step in the TF-CBT process, laying the groundwork for effective and tailored interventions. By taking the time to thoroughly assess, understand, and collaborate, you set the stage for meaningful change and healing. Remember, each client brings their own unique story and experiences, and your role is to help them rewrite that story, transforming pain into resilience and hope. As you move forward in this journey, keep in mind the importance of flexibility and adaptability, as the treatment plan may evolve as new insights and challenges arise. Now, let's continue on this path, equipped with a solid foundation and a shared understanding, as we explore the therapeutic techniques and interventions that will facilitate healing and growth.

.

Part II

Therapeutic Techniques for Trauma:

Psychoeducation and Skills Building

Psychoeducation and skills building form the foundation of trauma-focused cognitive-behavioral therapy (TF-CBT). This is where we lay the groundwork for healing by enhancing our clients' understanding of trauma and its effects and equipping them with a toolkit of coping strategies. By improving their knowledge and skills, we empower them to actively participate in their recovery journey and build resilience against future challenges.

Let's begin by exploring the concept of psychoeducation and why it's crucial in TF-CT. When someone has experienced trauma, their world can feel confusing and overwhelming. They might struggle to make sense of their thoughts, emotions, and behaviors, especially if they are experiencing symptoms of post-traumatic stress disorder (**PTSD**) or other trauma-related disorders. Psychoeducation helps shine a light on these confusing experiences and provides a framework for understanding them.

During psychoeducation sessions, we gently guide our clients through the basics of trauma and its impact on the brain and body. We explain how trauma can disrupt normal stress responses, leading to symptoms like hyperarousal, re-experiencing, or dissociation. By normalizing these reactions and providing a scientific context, we help reduce shame and self-blame while fostering a sense of validation and self-compassion.

For example, imagine a young girl named Emily who witnessed a car accident and now experiences panic attacks and flashbacks. Through psychoeducation, we can help Emily understand that her body's automatic survival responses, though frightening, are entirely normal reactions to an abnormal event. We can explain how trauma can sometimes overload the brain's alarm system, leading to heightened anxiety or sudden emotional outbursts. By learning about the fight-flight-freeze response and the role of stress hormones, Emily can begin to make sense of her symptoms and feel more in control.

Trauma triggers are another important topic to cover. Triggers are stimuli that remind individuals of their traumatic experiences and can elicit intense emotional or physical reactions. Together with our clients, we can explore common triggers, such as specific sights, sounds, smells, or even certain emotions or sensations. For instance, the sound of a car backfiring might trigger flashbacks to a shooting incident. By identifying these triggers, we can develop strategies to manage them effectively, reducing their impact and helping our clients feel safer in their environment.

Coping strategies are the cornerstone of skills building. Here, we teach our clients a variety of techniques to manage their trauma symptoms and improve emotional regulation. Deep breathing exercises, progressive muscle relaxation, and guided visualizations can all help calm the nervous system and promote a sense of tranquility. Mindfulness practices, such as grounding techniques or mindful movement, can also enhance present-moment awareness and reduce dissociation.

Let's introduce Emily to the concept of a 'calm anchor.' This involves teaching her a simple deep breathing exercise that she can use whenever she feels anxious or overwhelmed. We might provide her with a worksheet that explains the steps of deep breathing and includes a relaxing visualization. For example, we could ask her to imagine herself in a peaceful forest, taking in the fresh scent of pine trees with each inhalation and releasing tension with each exhalation. With regular practice, Emily can develop her own 'calm anchor' to access whenever she needs to steady herself during turbulent times.

Another valuable skill is emotional regulation. Trauma can disrupt individuals' ability to manage their emotions effectively, leading to intense or unpredictable mood swings. We can teach our clients to identify their emotions accurately and then offer a range of strategies to cope with difficult feelings. This might include creating an 'emotion toolkit' with different techniques, such as journaling, drawing or painting emotions, practicing assertive communication, or engaging in enjoyable physical activities to release pent-up emotions.

For instance, if Emily tends to internalize her emotions and struggles with self-expression, we could introduce her to the 'feelings thermometer.' This simple visual tool helps her identify the intensity of her emotions on a scale of 1 to 10 and then offers corresponding strategies for each level. At a level 3, she might simply need to take a few deep breaths, while at a level 8, she might benefit from going for a run or punching a pillow to release the pent-up energy.

The beauty of these skills is that they are portable and can be practiced anywhere, anytime. They become like tools in a toolkit that our clients can draw upon whenever they need to manage challenging symptoms or situations. By regularly practicing these coping strategies, individuals can improve their emotional resilience and feel more equipped to handle trauma triggers and stressful events.

In addition to relaxation and emotional regulation techniques, it's important to address common cognitive distortions associated with trauma. Negative thought patterns, such as all-or-nothing thinking or catastrophizing, can fuel anxiety and depression. We can provide worksheets and exercises to help our clients identify and challenge these unhelpful thoughts, encouraging a more balanced perspective.

For example, we might introduce the concept of 'thought challenging' and provide a thought record worksheet. This tool prompts individuals to identify triggering situations, the resulting negative thoughts, and then generate more realistic and helpful alternative thoughts. By doing so, they can gradually shift their thinking patterns and improve their overall mood and self-talk.

The psychoeducation and skills-building phase is a collaborative process, and it's important to tailor the content to the client's specific needs, age, and cultural background. We might incorporate creative activities, such as art, music, or drama, to make the learning experience more engaging and accessible. Additionally, involving caregivers or support systems can enhance the generalization of skills outside the therapy room.

By investing time in psychoeducation and skills building, we provide our clients with a solid foundation for the rest of their therapeutic journey. These tools not only help manage trauma symptoms but also foster a sense of agency and hope. As they continue through the TF-CBT process, they will build upon this foundation, gradually confronting traumatic memories and reshaping their relationship with their past experiences.

Remember, the ultimate goal is to empower our clients to become their own therapists, equipped with the knowledge and skills to navigate life's challenges and embrace a brighter, more resilient future.

Trauma Processing and Cognitive Restructuring

Trauma processing and cognitive restructuring are integral components of trauma-focused cognitive-behavioral therapy (CBT). These techniques enable individuals to confront and reshape their traumatic memories, thoughts, and beliefs, ultimately reducing the power these experiences hold over their lives. In this section, we will delve into the world of trauma processing, exploring three primary approaches: imaginal exposure, cognitive processing therapy, and narrative therapy. We will also discuss cognitive restructuring as a tool to challenge and transform negative thought patterns that often accompany trauma. By the end of this section, you should have a comprehensive understanding of these therapeutic techniques and their potential applications when working with trauma-exposed girls.

Trauma processing is a therapeutic journey that involves revisiting and re-experiencing traumatic memories in a safe and controlled manner. This process aims to reduce the intense emotional and physiological reactions associated with the trauma, allowing individuals to integrate these experiences into their narrative in a healthier way. One effective approach to trauma processing is imaginal exposure. With this technique, clients are guided to imagine and describe their traumatic memory in detail, gradually and repeatedly, until the memory loses its emotional charge. By facing their fears and approaching traumatic content head-on, clients can develop a sense of mastery and control over their reactions. For example, a girl who experienced a car accident might be asked to imagine the scene, the sounds, and her feelings during the event, gradually decreasing her fear response and helping her process the trauma.

Cognitive Processing Therapy (CPT) is another powerful tool in our trauma-focused CBT arsenal. CPT focuses on challenging and modifying dysfunctional thoughts and beliefs that arise from traumatic experiences. Individuals are encouraged to identify and explore their negative cognitions, evaluate the evidence for and against these thoughts, and develop more balanced and realistic alternatives. For instance, a common belief among trauma survivors is "I am unsafe," which can lead to heightened anxiety and avoidance behaviors. Through CPT, a client might examine the evidence for this belief, recognize that not all situations are inherently dangerous, and develop a more adaptive thought, such as "I can take steps to ensure my safety."

Narrative therapy offers a unique perspective on trauma processing by externalizing the problem. This approach views traumatic experiences as separate from the individual's core identity. Clients are encouraged to co-create a narrative or story about their trauma, often using metaphor and symbolism. By distancing themselves from the trauma and viewing it as a part of their life story rather than their entire identity, individuals can gain a sense of agency and begin to rewrite their narrative in a more empowering way. For example, a girl who experienced bullying might create a narrative where she is the protagonist facing a challenging obstacle, ultimately emerging stronger and more resilient.

Cognitive restructuring is a vital aspect of trauma-focused CBT, addressing the negative thought patterns and beliefs that often arise after trauma. These unhelpful thoughts can maintain or exacerbate distress, impacting an individual's mood, behavior, and overall functioning. The goal of cognitive restructuring is to identify, challenge, and replace these negative cognitions with more realistic and adaptive thoughts. For instance, a common negative thought among trauma survivors is "It was my fault," leading to feelings of guilt and shame. Cognitive restructuring would involve examining the evidence for this thought, recognizing external factors and the role of the perpetrator(s), and reframing it to "It was not my fault; I was a victim of circumstances beyond my control."

The process of cognitive restructuring typically involves several steps. First, therapists help clients identify and become aware of their negative thought patterns through techniques like thought recording or journaling. Next, they collaborate to challenge these thoughts by examining the evidence and considering alternative explanations. Then, they work together to generate more balanced and helpful thoughts, focusing on reality-testing and personal validation. Finally, clients are encouraged to practice implementing these new thoughts in their daily lives, gradually shifting their belief systems and emotional responses.

It is important to note that trauma processing and cognitive restructuring can evoke strong emotions and reactions. Therapists must ensure a strong therapeutic alliance and provide ample support and grounding techniques to help clients manage any distress. These techniques should be used within a safe and controlled therapeutic environment, gradually exposing clients to traumatic content and providing resources to cope with any emotional fallout. Additionally, it is crucial to assess each client's readiness for trauma processing, as attempting these techniques too early or without adequate preparation can be counterproductive.

Trauma processing and cognitive restructuring are powerful tools in our therapeutic toolbox, offering a pathway to healing and recovery for trauma survivors. By guiding individuals to confront and reshape their traumatic memories and thoughts, we empower them to rewrite their narrative and reclaim their lives. As therapists, it is our duty to skillfully and compassionately facilitate this journey, ensuring a sense of safety, support, and empowerment throughout the process.

Behavioral Activation and Experiential Techniques

Behavioral activation is a therapeutic approach rooted in the idea that our behaviors have a significant impact on our thoughts and emotions. When individuals experience trauma, they often develop avoidance behaviors as a way to cope with difficult thoughts, memories, or situations. While avoidance may provide temporary relief, it reinforces a cycle of fear and anxiety, maintaining the power that trauma holds over their lives.

The goal of behavioral activation is to help clients increase their engagement in values-driven actions, even when they feel challenging or scary. By taking small, manageable steps toward valued goals, clients can begin to break the cycle of avoidance and reclaim a sense of control. This approach aligns closely with trauma-focused CBT, as it emphasizes facing fears and challenging unhelpful behaviors in a gradual and supportive manner.

A critical first step in behavioral activation is helping clients identify their core values – the guiding principles that give their lives meaning and purpose. Values may include relationships, health, personal growth, creativity, or community contribution. By clarifying these values, clients can set meaningful goals that are intrinsically motivating. For example, a client may value family connections, so a goal could be to rebuild trust and improve communication with a parent.

Therapists can guide clients in setting specific, measurable, achievable, relevant, and time-bound (SMART) goals that align with their values. Using the previous example, a SMART goal could be to have an open and honest conversation with their parent about their trauma, taking a vulnerable yet courageous step toward repairing their relationship. This goal is rooted in the client's value of family connections and provides a tangible direction for their therapeutic journey.

Trauma-Related Exposure Exercises

Exposure exercises are a crucial aspect of behavioral activation in the context of trauma-focused CBT. These exercises involve gradually and safely confronting trauma-related memories, thoughts, or situations that the client has been avoiding. Exposure helps individuals process their traumatic experiences, reduce fear responses, and challenge unhelpful beliefs associated with the trauma.

Exposure exercises can take various forms, such as imaginal exposure, where clients visualize and narrate their traumatic memories, or in vivo exposure, where they confront feared situations or objects in real-life settings. For example, a client who experienced a car accident may start by imagining themselves driving again, gradually working up to actually getting behind the wheel and eventually driving on the highway.

Experiential Techniques: Bringing Healing to Life

While cognitive and behavioral strategies are essential, the inclusion of experiential techniques adds a powerful dimension to the therapeutic process. These techniques provide opportunities for clients to actively engage their senses and bodies in the healing process, often revealing insights and emotions that words alone may not access.

Role-Playing

Role-playing is a valuable experiential technique that allows clients to practice new behaviors, assertiveness, or communication skills in a safe and controlled environment. Therapists can guide clients through role-playing scenarios relevant to their trauma, such as setting boundaries, expressing emotions, or navigating challenging conversations. This technique helps clients build confidence and prepare for similar situations they may encounter in their daily lives.

Art Therapy

Art therapy offers a non-verbal mode of expression that can be particularly beneficial for clients who struggle to articulate their thoughts and emotions. Through drawing, painting, collaging, or sculpting, clients can externalize their internal experiences and gain new perspectives. Art therapy provides a means to symbolically express trauma, process difficult emotions, and foster self-soothing. For example, a client may create a collage representing their trauma and recovery journey, incorporating images that symbolize their pain, strength, and hope.

Somatic Experiencing

Somatic experiencing is an approach that focuses on the mind-body connection, recognizing that trauma is stored not only in memories but also in the body's physiological responses. This technique helps clients notice and regulate their physical sensations, such as rapid heartbeat, muscle tension, or shallow breathing. By tracking and gently releasing these sensations, clients can learn to discharge trapped energy and cultivate a sense of safety and grounding in their bodies.

Overcoming Obstacles and Building Momentum

Initiating behavioral changes and confronting trauma-related experiences can be daunting for clients. It's essential to acknowledge and address common obstacles, such as fear of triggering emotions, lack of motivation, or self-doubt. Therapists can support clients in developing strategies to overcome these challenges, such as breaking tasks into smaller steps, utilizing coping skills, and celebrating even the smallest successes.

To build momentum, therapists can also encourage clients to reflect on their values and the benefits of taking action. Highlighting the progress made and reinforcing the sense of accomplishment can be motivating. Additionally, connecting clients with support systems or peer groups can provide accountability and a sense of community during this transformative process.

Integrating Behavioral Activation into Therapy

Behavioral activation is most effective when tailored to the individual's unique needs and goals. Therapists can incorporate behavioral strategies throughout the therapeutic process, starting with small, manageable actions and gradually increasing the level of challenge. It's important to assess the client's comfort level and pace the introduction of exposure exercises accordingly, ensuring a sense of safety and control.

By combining behavioral activation with the other components of trauma-focused CBT, therapists can facilitate comprehensive healing. As clients engage in values-based actions and confront trauma-related experiences, they can process underlying thoughts and emotions, challenge unhelpful beliefs, and cultivate resilience.

Behavioral activation and experiential techniques provide the framework for clients to actively engage in their healing journey. Through values-driven actions, exposure exercises, and creative modalities, individuals can reclaim their power, challenge trauma-related fears, and rebuild a life rooted in courage and authenticity. As therapists, we bear witness to their transformative process, supporting and guiding them toward a brighter future unshackled by the constraints of trauma.

Addressing Common Trauma Responses

As a therapist working with trauma-exposed girls, you'll often encounter a range of emotional and behavioral responses that can significantly impact their lives. Understanding and effectively managing these common trauma responses are crucial steps in the healing process. In this section, we'll delve into some of the most prevalent reactions to trauma and explore strategies within the framework of trauma-focused CBT to help your clients navigate these challenging emotions and behaviors.

Anxiety and Fear:

Trauma often leaves individuals with a heightened sense of anxiety and fear. They may find themselves on constant alert, anticipating danger even in safe environments. This "fight-or-flight" response can manifest as excessive worrying, difficulty concentrating, restlessness, or physical symptoms like rapid heartbeat or sweating. To help manage anxiety, educate your clients about the mind-body connection and how trauma can disrupt the body's natural alarm system. Teach relaxation techniques such as deep breathing, progressive muscle relaxation, or guided visualizations to help them calm their nervous system and cultivate a sense of safety and control. Encourage your clients to identify and challenge anxious thoughts using cognitive restructuring techniques. For example, they can learn to recognize catastrophic thinking ("Something terrible is going to happen") and replace it with more realistic and adaptive thoughts ("I am safe right now, and I can handle difficult situations").

Additionally, gradual exposure therapy can be incredibly beneficial. Start by creating a fear hierarchy, a ladder of feared situations ranked from least to most anxiety-provoking. Begin with milder fears and use coping strategies to navigate through them successfully. Gradually move up the hierarchy, helping your clients face their fears in a safe and controlled manner. This process helps rewrite the brain's response to feared stimuli and builds resilience.

Depression and Emotional Numbness:

Trauma can often lead to feelings of overwhelming sadness, hopelessness, and a loss of interest in previously enjoyable activities—signaling depression. Some individuals may also experience emotional numbness, feeling detached from their emotions and the world around them. To address these responses, it's crucial to help your clients identify and process their emotions effectively. Encourage them to keep a journal to express their feelings, thoughts, and experiences. Writing can be a powerful tool for externalizing emotions and making sense of traumatic events. Engage your clients in activities that foster a sense of pleasure or accomplishment, even if it's a small step, to help lift their mood and rebuild motivation.

Trauma-focused CBT can also help challenge negative thought patterns associated with depression. Identify and challenge unhelpful beliefs, such as "I am worthless" or "nothing will ever change." Replace these with more balanced and positive thoughts, like "I am valuable and deserving of love" or "change is possible, and I can take small steps towards a brighter future." Behavioral activation is another effective strategy, encouraging your clients to engage in activities that bring a sense of fulfillment or accomplishment, even when they don't feel like it.

Anger and Irritability:

Anger is a common response to trauma, often serving as a protective emotion that masks underlying pain, fear, or vulnerability. However, when anger becomes intense, frequent, or difficult to control, it can negatively impact relationships and daily functioning. To help your clients manage anger, start by validating their right to feel angry and acknowledging the underlying emotions that anger may disguise. Teach anger management techniques, such as deep breathing, counting to ten, or taking a "time-out" when anger escalates. Encourage your clients to identify anger triggers and develop healthy coping strategies, such as exercising, journaling, or engaging in creative outlets like art or music.

Exploring the underlying causes of anger is essential. Use trauma-focused CBT techniques to identify and challenge angry thoughts, such as "They did this to me on purpose" or "I must get revenge." Help your clients understand how these thoughts contribute to their anger and guide them toward more realistic and less inflammatory interpretations. Role-playing and rehearsal can also be useful, helping your clients practice assertiveness and effective communication skills to express their needs and set boundaries in a healthy manner.

Shame and Self-Blame:

Shame is a pervasive and debilitating emotion that often arises after trauma, leading individuals to believe they are flawed, unworthy, or somehow responsible for what happened. To address shame, it's crucial to create a safe and non-judgmental therapeutic environment. Help your clients understand that shame is a normal response to trauma but an inaccurate reflection of their self-worth. Encourage self-compassion and self-acceptance by practicing self-soothing techniques and positive self-talk. Writing a letter to oneself from the perspective of a compassionate other can also help challenge self-critical thoughts and cultivate self-compassion.

Trauma-focused CBT can be particularly effective in reframing self-blaming thoughts and beliefs. Guide your clients in identifying and disputing self-blaming statements, such as "It's my fault this happened" or "I should have done something to prevent it." Help them understand the role of perpetrators and external factors, shifting the blame away from themselves. Exploring personal values and strengths can also help rebuild self-worth and challenge shame-based beliefs.

Self-Harm and Risky Behaviors:

Trauma can sometimes lead individuals to engage in self-harm or risky behaviors as a means of coping with overwhelming emotions or feeling in control. It's important to address these behaviors directly and safely. Help your clients understand the underlying causes and triggers for their self-harm or risky behaviors. Encourage them to develop safer coping strategies, such as using a rubber band to snap against the wrist, holding ice, or engaging in intense exercise. Explore alternative ways to manage emotions, such as through emotional regulation skills or distress tolerance techniques.

For clients engaging in self-harm, it's crucial to assess the severity and frequency of the behavior and determine if higher levels of care or crisis intervention are necessary. Collaborate with your clients to develop a safety plan, identifying triggers, coping strategies, and sources of support to help them manage urges and stay safe. Addressing underlying emotional distress and trauma through trauma-focused CBT can also help reduce the compulsion to self-harm.

Trauma can evoke a myriad of responses, and it's important to remember that each individual's experience is unique. By understanding and addressing these common trauma responses—anxiety, depression, anger, shame, and self-harm—within the framework of trauma-focused CBT, you can empower your clients to manage their emotions effectively, challenge unhelpful thoughts, and develop healthier coping strategies. Always adapt your approach to meet the specific needs of each client, drawing from a range of therapeutic techniques to facilitate their healing journey. Remember, healing is a process, and with your guidance, trauma survivors can reclaim their lives and embrace a brighter future.

Part III

Working with Specific Populations:

Trauma in Childhood and Adolescence

Working with trauma in childhood and adolescence presents unique challenges and considerations. The impact of trauma during these formative years can have profound and lasting effects on a person's development, emotions, and behavior. In this section, we will delve into the intricate world of trauma as it relates to young people, exploring the various types of trauma they may encounter and how it manifests across different age groups. We will also discuss trauma-informed parenting strategies, offering guidance to caregivers who play a crucial role in the healing process.

Trauma in childhood and adolescence can take many forms. It may result from a single traumatic event, such as a natural disaster, a violent attack, or a serious accident. However, it is important to recognize that trauma can also arise from ongoing and pervasive adverse experiences. This includes situations like chronic illness, living in a war zone, or enduring sustained emotional abuse or neglect. Understanding the diverse nature of trauma is essential when working with young people, as it shapes their perspective, behaviors, and overall functioning.

Developmental Considerations

The impact of trauma on a child or adolescent varies depending on their developmental stage. Let's explore how trauma presents and how we can intervene effectively at different ages:

Early Childhood (Ages 3 to 6)

In early childhood, trauma often disrupts the formation of secure attachments and can lead to significant challenges in emotional regulation and social interactions. Young children may exhibit regressive behaviors, increased clinginess, or difficulty separating from caregivers. They might struggle with fear, anxiety, and disruptive behaviors. Therapeutic interventions at this age often involve supporting the caregiver-child relationship, promoting safety and stability, and teaching simple coping strategies like deep breathing or using calming sensory objects. Play therapy can be incredibly beneficial, as it allows children to process their experiences through a natural and developmentally appropriate medium.

Middle Childhood (Ages 6 to 12)

During middle childhood, trauma can interfere with the development of self-esteem, academic skills, and peer relationships. Children in this age group may exhibit symptoms of anxiety and depression, act out aggressively, or withdraw socially. They might struggle with concentration and experience learning difficulties. Interventions often focus on psychoeducation, helping them understand and label their emotions. Teaching concrete coping strategies, such as grounding techniques or positive self-talk, can be very effective. Encouraging participation in structured activities and fostering social connections through group therapy or peer support can also promote healing.

Adolescence (Ages 13 to 18)

Trauma in adolescence can have a profound impact on identity formation, emotional regulation, and decision-making. Teenagers may exhibit risk-taking behaviors, substance use, self-harm, or suicidal ideation. They might struggle with trust issues, rebellion, or a sense of isolation. Therapeutic interventions often involve helping adolescents develop emotional awareness and healthy coping mechanisms. Exploring their sense of self and fostering resilience through strengths-based approaches is crucial. Group therapy can be particularly beneficial during this stage, as it provides a sense of belonging and allows for peer support and normalization.

Attachment Trauma and Complex Trauma

When working with trauma in childhood and adolescence, it is essential to recognize the prevalence of attachment trauma and complex trauma. Attachment trauma occurs when a child's primary caregiver, typically a source of safety and security, becomes a source of fear or instability due to abuse, neglect, or inconsistent caregiving. This can lead to significant disturbances in the child's ability to form secure attachments and regulate their emotions effectively. Complex trauma, also known as developmental trauma, arises from prolonged and repeated exposure to traumatic events, often involving multiple types of trauma and ongoing adversity. It can result in pervasive negative effects on the child's sense of self, relationships, and functioning across various life domains.

Addressing attachment trauma and complex trauma requires a comprehensive and nuanced approach. Therapists should focus on rebuilding trust, promoting emotional safety, and strengthening secure attachments. This may involve working closely with caregivers to enhance their understanding of trauma and its impact on attachment patterns. Caregivers can be guided to provide consistent, responsive, and nurturing care, helping their children feel safe, loved, and supported.

Trauma-Informed Parenting Strategies

Involving caregivers in the healing process is crucial, as they play a pivotal role in creating a trauma-informed environment that supports their child's recovery. Here are some key strategies to guide caregivers:

- **Safety and Stability:** Emphasize the importance of establishing a safe and stable home environment, free from violence, substance abuse, or other adverse factors. Consistency and predictability in daily routines can also promote a sense of security.

- **Responsive Caregiving:** Encourage caregivers to be attuned to their child's emotional and physical needs, offering comfort, validation, and support. Teaching caregivers about the impact of trauma on their child's development can enhance their responsiveness.

- **Positive Discipline:** Guide caregivers toward using positive discipline strategies that focus on teaching and redirection rather than punishment. This helps children learn self-regulation and promotes a sense of cooperation.

- **Self-Care and Regulation:** Educate caregivers about the importance of their self-care and modeling healthy emotional regulation. When caregivers can manage their own emotions effectively, they can better support their children in doing the same.

- **Trauma-Sensitive Communication:** Encourage open and honest communication, creating a safe space for children to express their feelings and experiences. Teach caregivers to listen non-judgmentally and validate their child's emotions.

- **Support Systems:** Help caregivers build their support network, whether through therapy, support groups, or community resources. Connecting with others who understand the impact of trauma can provide valuable guidance and reduce feelings of isolation.

Working with trauma in childhood and adolescence is a delicate and complex process. By recognizing the unique developmental considerations, addressing attachment trauma and complex trauma, and involving caregivers in trauma-informed parenting strategies, we can foster healing and resilience in young people. It is through this comprehensive approach that we can support them in reclaiming their lives and reaching their full potential.

As therapists and caregivers, we have the privilege and responsibility to walk alongside these brave individuals, offering guidance, compassion, and hope as they navigate the path toward healing and a brighter future.

Intersectionality and Cultural Competence

As we delve into the intricate interplay between trauma and identity, it's essential to recognize that trauma doesn't occur in a vacuum. It intersects with various aspects of an individual's life, including their gender, race, ethnicity, sexual orientation, socio-economic status, and other social identities. This section explores the concept of intersectionality and its profound implications for trauma-informed therapy. We will also delve into cultural competence, emphasizing the importance of adapting trauma-focused CBT to meet the diverse needs of our clients. By embracing a culturally sensitive and inclusive approach, we can more effectively support healing and resilience in all communities.

Understanding Intersectionality

At the heart of intersectionality is the recognition that our identities are multifaceted and interconnected. When it comes to trauma, these identities can shape an individual's experiences, both in terms of their vulnerability to trauma and their journey towards healing. For example, a young girl from a racial minority group may face not only the trauma of sexual abuse but also the additional layers of discrimination and systemic racism, impacting her access to support and shaping her overall well-being.

Trauma can exacerbate existing inequalities and marginalization, and it's crucial for therapists to understand how these factors interplay. By acknowledging and addressing the unique challenges faced by diverse populations, we can provide more holistic and effective care. This section will delve into the specific ways trauma intersects with different identities, shedding light on the nuanced experiences of individuals from various backgrounds.

Trauma and Gender

While this book primarily focuses on trauma in girls and women, it's important to acknowledge that gender is a spectrum, and trauma can affect individuals across the gender spectrum in unique ways. For example, transgender and non-binary individuals may face trauma related to gender dysphoria, discrimination, or the lack of inclusive support systems. Therapists should be attuned to these specific challenges and create safe spaces that validate and honor the diverse gender identities of their clients.

Race, Ethnicity, and Cultural Backgrounds

The impact of racial trauma cannot be overstated. Individuals from racial and ethnic minority groups may face unique traumas related to discrimination, racial profiling, microaggressions, or historical trauma passed down through generations. Cultural backgrounds also play a significant role, influencing beliefs about mental health, help-seeking behaviors, and the expression of emotional distress. Therapists must be aware of their own cultural lens and actively work to understand the cultural context of their clients' experiences.

Sexual Orientation and Gender Diversity

LGBTQIA+ individuals may encounter trauma related to discrimination, rejection, or internalized homophobia and transphobia. The coming-out process, family rejection, and experiences of bullying or violence can all contribute to trauma. Therapists should create safe and affirming spaces, recognizing the unique challenges and strengths of LGBTQIA+ individuals and communities.

Socio-Economic Status and Education

Trauma knows no socio-economic boundaries, but individuals from low-income backgrounds may face additional barriers to healing. Limited access to mental health services, stigma surrounding mental illness, and the daily stressors of poverty can complicate the recovery process. Education also plays a role, as trauma can interfere with learning and academic achievement, impacting an individual's future opportunities.

Immigration Status and Refugee Experiences

The trauma of displacement, separation from loved ones, and the challenges of adapting to a new culture are unique to immigrants and refugees. Language barriers, acculturative stress, and the potential retraumatization from reminders of past trauma in a new environment can complicate the healing process. Therapists should be mindful of these factors and incorporate cultural humility into their practice.

Disability and Trauma

Individuals with disabilities may face trauma related to ableism, accessibility barriers, or the medical model of disability, which focuses on "fixing" rather than accommodating. The additional layer of trauma can exacerbate existing challenges and impact an individual's sense of self-worth. Therapists should embrace a strengths-based approach, recognizing the resilience and capabilities of individuals with disabilities.

Cultural Competence in Therapy

Cultural competence is about more than just understanding cultural differences; it's a commitment to ongoing self-reflection, learning, and adaptation. As therapists, we must recognize our own cultural lenses and biases and actively work to provide culturally responsive care. This includes being open to feedback, seeking supervision or consultation when needed, and continually educating ourselves about diverse cultures and communities.

Adapting Trauma-Focused CBT for Diverse Populations

While trauma-focused CBT has been proven effective, it's not a one-size-fits-all approach. Adapting the framework to honor cultural differences is essential. This may involve incorporating cultural concepts of healing, such as traditional rituals or spiritual practices, into the therapeutic process. It also means being mindful of language and communication styles, ensuring that interventions are accessible and culturally relevant.

For example, when working with Indigenous communities, therapists can integrate traditional healing practices, such as smudging or talking circles, into CBT techniques. Collaborating with cultural elders or community leaders can help ensure that interventions are culturally safe and respectful. Similarly, when working with individuals from collectivist cultures, involving family or community members in the therapeutic process may be beneficial, provided it aligns with the client's wishes and cultural norms.

Building Inclusive Spaces

Creating inclusive therapy spaces is crucial to fostering trust and engagement. This includes using inclusive language, avoiding assumptions, and actively addressing power dynamics. Therapists should be mindful of their office environment, ensuring that it reflects diversity and cultural sensitivity. This may involve displaying diverse artwork, offering a variety of reading materials in the waiting room, or playing music from different cultural backgrounds.

Community Collaboration and Advocacy

Cultural competence extends beyond the therapy room. Therapists can actively engage in community collaboration and advocacy to address systemic inequalities and promote trauma-informed practices on a broader scale. This may involve partnering with community organizations, participating in cultural events, or advocating for policy changes that support trauma-informed approaches in schools, healthcare settings, and the justice system.

Cultural competence is a lifelong journey. Therapists should continually seek out educational opportunities, whether through workshops, webinars, or reading diverse literature. Engaging in self-reflection and seeking feedback from colleagues and clients is also essential. By embracing a growth mindset, we can continually enhance our cultural responsiveness and better serve our diverse clients.

As we conclude this section, it's important to recognize that intersectionality and cultural competence are not optional add-ons to our therapeutic practice; they are fundamental to providing effective and ethical care. By embracing diversity and adapting our approaches to meet the unique needs of each client, we honor their resilience and empower them on their healing journey. Let us continue to challenge ourselves, expand our understanding, and create safe and inclusive spaces for all individuals impacted by trauma. Together, we can foster a more equitable and trauma-responsive society.

Trauma in High-Risk Populations

It's important to recognize that trauma knows no boundaries and can infiltrate the lives of individuals from all walks of life. Yet, there are certain populations that bear the brunt of trauma's relentless grip more intensely. These are the survivors who have endured unimaginable hardships, often facing a multitude of traumas that intertwine and compound one another. They are the survivors of abuse, the victims of human trafficking, and those who have borne witness to relentless community violence. Their stories are not for the faint of heart, but they are a testament to the resilience of the human spirit. As we navigate these complex paths to healing, it's crucial to approach these high-risk populations with a nuanced understanding and an arsenal of tailored strategies.

Survivors of Abuse: Unraveling the Threads of Trauma

For survivors of abuse, the very fabric of trust and safety has been torn apart. Whether it's the insidious violation of emotional abuse, the haunting shadows of sexual abuse, or the visible scars of physical abuse, the impact can be profound and far-reaching. Often, abuse occurs within the very places that should offer sanctuary – homes, schools, or religious institutions. This betrayal of trust can leave survivors struggling with complex trauma, where the wounds of the past seep into every facet of their present lives.

When working with survivors of abuse, it's imperative to create a safe and non-judgmental space where they can begin to unravel their painful experiences. This often involves addressing issues of shame and self-blame, as survivors may internalize the abuse and question their self-worth. Techniques such as cognitive restructuring can help challenge these negative core beliefs and rewrite the narrative of self-blame into one of empowerment and self-compassion. Additionally, trauma-focused CBT can assist survivors in processing specific traumatic events, allowing them to confront and reframe the memories that haunt them.

For these survivors, rebuilding trust and establishing healthy boundaries are essential aspects of recovery. Therapists can guide them in recognizing unhealthy patterns in relationships and empower them to set clear and assertive boundaries. Role-playing exercises can be particularly useful in practicing these skills. Furthermore, survivors of abuse often benefit from exploring their support systems and expanding their social networks. Encouraging them to seek out support groups or peer support can provide a sense of connection and validation.

Human Trafficking Survivors: Unshackling the Chains of Trauma

Human trafficking, a modern form of slavery, inflicts trauma on a profound scale. The very essence of a person's autonomy and freedom is stripped away, leaving deep scars that extend beyond physical injuries. Survivors often endure prolonged periods of captivity, exploitation, and unimaginable abuse. The trauma they experience is complex and layered, encompassing physical, sexual, and psychological abuse, as well as severe violations of human rights.

The journey of healing for human trafficking survivors is a delicate and intricate process. It requires addressing the immediate needs for safety and stabilization, followed by a comprehensive trauma-focused approach. This may involve helping survivors regain a sense of control and agency over their lives, as traffickers often use manipulation and coercion to exert power. Therapists can assist survivors in identifying and challenging the negative beliefs and self-perceptions that may have been instilled during their exploitation.

Given the extensive control and isolation tactics employed by traffickers, it's crucial to help survivors rebuild their sense of self and identity. Exploring their interests, values, and aspirations can be a powerful step in this direction. Additionally, practical support is essential, including assistance with legal matters, housing, and employment. Connecting survivors with specialized anti-trafficking organizations and survivor support networks can provide them with a community of support and a sense of belonging.

Community Violence: Navigating a World of Unrelenting Trauma

Community violence casts a wide net, ensnaring individuals, families, and entire neighborhoods in its destructive path. From witnessing gang-related shootings to experiencing the pervasive fear of domestic terrorism, the impact of community violence reaches far beyond those directly involved. The relentless exposure to violence becomes a pervasive trauma, shaping the lives of children, adolescents, and adults alike.

For individuals impacted by community violence, the sense of safety and security in their environment is shattered. They may struggle with constant fear, hypervigilance, and a heightened sense of danger. Trauma-focused CBT can help process specific traumatic events, such as witnessing a shooting or surviving a violent attack. Additionally, addressing trauma responses like anxiety, anger, or substance use becomes crucial in fostering resilience and preventing the intergenerational transmission of trauma.

Given the pervasive nature of community violence, a multi-faceted approach is necessary. This includes individual therapy, but also extends to community-based interventions. Collaborating with local organizations, schools, and faith-based groups can create a network of support. Educating communities about trauma and its impact can foster a collective understanding and promote healing on a broader scale. Additionally, advocating for policy changes that address the root causes of community violence becomes an integral part of long-term prevention and healing.

Common Threads and Tailored Strategies:

As we explore these distinct yet interconnected high-risk populations, certain commonalities emerge. First and foremost, the need for safety and stabilization takes precedence. This may involve connecting individuals to crisis intervention services, safe housing, or legal advocacy. Practical support is often a critical first step in establishing a foundation for healing.

Secondly, the intricate dance between trauma processing and skill-building comes into play. Trauma-focused CBT provides a framework for processing traumatic memories and challenging negative cognitions. Simultaneously, teaching coping strategies, such as relaxation techniques, emotional regulation skills, and distress tolerance, becomes essential for managing trauma responses.

For these populations, the therapeutic relationship itself can be a powerful agent of change. Establishing trust, empathy, and a sense of collaboration are key. Therapists must be attuned to potential power dynamics and work to empower survivors, offering choices and a sense of control within the therapeutic process.

Lastly, the journey of healing extends beyond the therapy room. Connecting survivors to additional resources, support groups, and peer networks can provide a sense of community and validation. Whether it's specialized organizations supporting survivors of human trafficking or community-based initiatives addressing the aftermath of violence, these resources offer a lifeline and a sense of belonging.

As we navigate the complexities of trauma in these high-risk populations, it's crucial to recognize the resilience and strength that lie within each survivor. They have weathered storms that most can barely fathom. Our role as therapists and allies is to shine a light on their path, offering guidance, support, and the tools necessary to reclaim their lives and forge a future unshackled by the chains of trauma.

In closing, let us carry the weight of these stories with reverence and resolve. May they fuel our determination to create a world where trauma is recognized, addressed, and ultimately prevented. Together, we can weave a tapestry of healing, where every survivor finds their voice, their strength, and their unique path to recovery.

Part IV

Clinical Applications and Special Considerations

Integrating Trauma-Focused CBT with Other Therapies

When working with younger children, integrating trauma-focused CBT with play therapy can be incredibly powerful. Play is a child's natural language, and it becomes a therapeutic tool to help them express themselves, process emotions, and make sense of their experiences. Within the context of play therapy, trauma-focused CBT techniques can be seamlessly woven into the child's play activities. For instance, a therapist might use cognitive restructuring to challenge negative thoughts through playful scenarios or utilize behavioral activation by encouraging the child to engage in enjoyable activities that promote a sense of mastery and resilience.

Consider a young girl who has experienced a traumatic event such as a car accident. Through play therapy, she can act out the scene using dolls or puppets, gradually processing the event and challenging any negative beliefs she may have developed, such as "I am not safe" or "bad things will keep happening." The therapist can gently guide the play to include coping strategies, such as the child's favorite stuffed animal offering comfort and support, modeling healthy ways to manage difficult emotions.

By incorporating play, therapists create a safe and non-threatening environment for children to explore their traumatic experiences. Play therapy techniques, such as role-playing, storytelling, or art-based activities, provide a means for children to externalize their thoughts and feelings, making them more accessible for examination and transformation. This integration allows young clients to process their trauma while simultaneously learning valuable skills to manage their emotions and behavior.

Family Therapy and Trauma-Focused CBT: A Collaborative Approach:

Trauma often impacts not just the individual but the entire family system. Integrating trauma-focused CBT with family therapy can facilitate healing not only for the survivor but for the family as a whole. Family therapy provides a unique perspective by addressing the dynamics, communication patterns, and relationships within the family unit, all of which can influence the trauma recovery process.

In family therapy sessions, trauma-focused CBT techniques can be adapted to involve the entire family. For example, during a session focused on cognitive restructuring, the therapist might engage the family in identifying and challenging negative thought patterns collectively. This could involve exploring how each family member interprets and responds to trauma-related behaviors, such as a child's withdrawal or irritability. Together, they can work on developing more adaptive thoughts and behaviors that promote understanding, support, and healthy family interactions.

Additionally, family therapy can be a platform for trauma education, helping family members understand the impact of trauma on brain development, attachment, and emotional regulation. This shared understanding fosters empathy, improves communication, and empowers family members to support each other effectively. The family becomes a source of strength and a vital part of the child's healing process, creating a cohesive and nurturing environment that extends beyond the therapy room.

The Mind-Body Connection: Trauma-Informed Yoga and CBT:

Trauma is held in the body as well as the mind, and integrating trauma-focused CBT with trauma-informed yoga offers a holistic approach to healing. Yoga provides an avenue for survivors to reconnect with their bodies, regulate their nervous systems, and develop a sense of embodiment. When combined with CBT, yoga becomes a powerful tool to enhance trauma processing and emotional resilience.

Trauma-informed yoga focuses on creating a safe and non-judgmental space, emphasizing choice and consent. Survivors are invited to notice and accept their physical and emotional sensations without judgment, a concept that aligns seamlessly with CBT's emphasis on mindfulness and present-moment awareness. As they move through yoga poses, survivors can begin to identify and tolerate intense emotions, practicing the skills of emotional regulation learned in CBT sessions.

For example, a survivor might notice feelings of anxiety arising during a balancing pose and recall CBT techniques to ground themselves in the present moment, such as focusing on the sensations of their feet firmly planted on the ground. The combination of CBT and yoga empowers individuals to develop a deeper sense of self-awareness, self-compassion, and self-efficacy, all of which contribute to their overall resilience and well-being.

Integrating these approaches can also provide survivors with a sense of agency and control over their recovery journey. They can actively choose to incorporate yoga into their self-care routines, enhancing the skills learned in therapy and extending the benefits beyond the therapist's office. The mind-body connection fostered through this integration promotes a more comprehensive and enduring healing process.

The integration of trauma-focused CBT with other therapeutic modalities is a testament to its flexibility and potential for innovation. Therapists can draw from a rich array of techniques, tailoring their interventions to meet the diverse needs of their clients. By blending these approaches, therapists create a comprehensive treatment plan that addresses the multifaceted nature of trauma and its impact on the individual.

For instance, consider the integration of trauma-focused CBT with expressive arts therapy, which includes modalities such as art, music, dance, or drama therapy. Creative expression can become a powerful vehicle for trauma survivors to externalize their experiences, providing a safe outlet for emotions that may be difficult to articulate through words alone. CBT techniques can be seamlessly woven into these expressive arts modalities, fostering insight, emotional release, and the development of adaptive coping strategies.

Similarly, the integration of trauma-focused CBT with mindfulness-based therapies, such as mindfulness-based stress reduction (MBSR) or dialectical behavior therapy (DBT), can enhance present-moment awareness, emotional regulation, and distress tolerance skills. Mindfulness practices, including mindful breathing, body scans, or walking meditations, can be incorporated into CBT sessions to ground survivors in the here and now, reducing the intensity of trauma-related symptoms and improving overall well-being.

The versatility of trauma-focused CBT extends beyond these examples, as it can be effectively integrated with other evidence-based therapies, including acceptance and commitment therapy (ACT), exposure and response prevention (ERP), or emotion-focused therapy (EFT). Each integration offers a unique perspective and set of tools to address the complex needs of trauma survivors, allowing therapists to create individualized treatment plans that resonate with their clients.

Trauma-focused CBT, with its structured framework and evidence-based foundation, provides a solid starting point for therapists working with trauma survivors. By integrating it with other therapeutic approaches, we expand our therapeutic toolbox, tailoring interventions to meet the diverse needs of our clients. Whether incorporating play therapy for younger clients, involving the entire family system, or exploring the mind-body connection through yoga, we enhance the healing process and empower survivors on their journey towards recovery.

As therapists, it is important to remain open to these integrative possibilities, continuously seeking training and education in complementary modalities. By embracing a collaborative and holistic approach, we honor the uniqueness of each client's journey and create a therapeutic alliance that fosters profound healing, growth, and transformation. Together, we can guide trauma survivors towards a brighter future, helping them reclaim their lives and discover a renewed sense of hope and resilience.

Working with Caregivers and Support Systems

Involving caregivers and support systems in the therapeutic process is an essential aspect of trauma-informed care. When a child or adolescent experiences trauma, the impact extends beyond the individual and reverberates through their relationships and support networks. Collaborating with caregivers and significant others not only enhances the effectiveness of trauma-focused CBT but also fosters a cohesive and supportive environment for the client's healing journey. In this chapter, we will delve into the intricate dynamics of engaging caregivers, offering guidance, and exploring strategies to navigate this crucial aspect of therapy.

Involving Caregivers in the Therapeutic Process:

When working with minors or young adults, it is imperative to recognize the pivotal role that caregivers play in their lives. Caregivers can be parents, guardians, foster parents, or any adult with a significant presence in the client's day-to-day life. Their involvement in therapy can take various forms, each contributing to the overall healing process:

- **Education and Awareness**: Educating caregivers about trauma and its effects is a fundamental step. Caregivers who understand the underlying causes of their loved one's behaviors, emotions, and symptoms can develop empathy and patience. Providing information about trauma responses, such as fight, flight, or freeze reactions, can help caregivers interpret their child's actions and reactions more accurately. Share resources, recommend books or articles, and encourage participation in support groups or educational workshops.

- **Collaborative Goal Setting**: Engaging caregivers in the goal-setting process fosters a sense of partnership and shared purpose. Invite caregivers to share their observations, concerns, and hopes for their child's therapy. Collaboratively establish goals that align with the client's needs and the caregiver's aspirations. For example, if a client is working on managing anger outbursts, the caregiver can be involved in setting goals for improved emotional regulation and identifying triggers within the home environment.

- **Consistent Communication**: Establish open and consistent communication channels with caregivers. Regular updates and progress reports help caregivers feel included and informed. Discuss the client's progress, challenges, and achievements. Share insights or strategies that caregivers can implement at home, reinforcing the therapeutic work. Remember to maintain confidentiality while sharing pertinent information that supports the client's treatment and well-being.

- **In-Session Participation:** Depending on the client's comfort level and therapeutic needs, consider inviting caregivers to participate in therapy sessions. This can take the form of joint sessions with the client and caregiver together or separate sessions specifically for the caregiver. In these sessions, you can explore the caregiver's experiences, address their questions or concerns, and provide skills training. Joint sessions can also be an opportunity for caregivers to learn how to support their child's coping strategies and practice effective communication skills.

Coping Strategies for Caregivers:

Supporting a loved one who has experienced trauma can be emotionally demanding and challenging. Caregivers may struggle with their own feelings of guilt, fear, or helplessness. Providing caregivers with concrete coping strategies can enhance their resilience and improve their ability to support the client effectively:

- **Self-Care Practices:** Emphasize the importance of self-care for caregivers. Encourage them to prioritize their physical and emotional well-being through practices such as regular exercise, healthy eating, and adequate sleep. Suggest relaxation techniques like deep breathing, meditation, or engaging in enjoyable hobbies and activities that provide a sense of replenishment.

- **Support Networks:** Encourage caregivers to build their support systems. Connect them with support groups specifically for caregivers of trauma survivors, where they can find understanding and shared experiences. Foster connections with other caregivers within the community or through online forums. These networks can provide a sense of community, validation, and practical advice.

- **Mindfulness and Emotional Regulation:** Teach caregivers mindfulness techniques to help them manage their own emotional responses. Guide them through practices such as mindful breathing, grounding exercises, or guided visualizations. Encourage caregivers to notice and acknowledge their feelings without judgment and explore strategies for effectively regulating their emotions.

- **Stress Management:** Provide stress management strategies tailored to caregivers' unique situations. This may include time management techniques, problem-solving skills, or identifying triggers for stress and developing healthy coping mechanisms. Encourage caregivers to set realistic expectations for themselves and practice self-compassion when facing challenges.

- **Education and Advocacy:** Empower caregivers with knowledge about trauma and its effects.

Provide resources and recommendations for further reading or online courses. Encourage them to become advocates for their loved one, understanding the impact of trauma on brain development, attachment, and behavior. Help them navigate the systems involved, such as the educational or legal system, and provide guidance on advocating for their child's needs.

Self-Care for Caregivers:

As caregivers dedicate themselves to supporting their loved one's healing journey, it is crucial that they also prioritize their self-care. Burnout, compassion fatigue, and secondary traumatic stress are real concerns for caregivers of trauma survivors. Helping caregivers recognize the signs of burnout and implementing proactive self-care strategies are essential for their well-being:

- **Recognizing Burnout:** Educate caregivers about the signs and symptoms of burnout, such as emotional exhaustion, depersonalization, decreased empathy, and physical or mental health issues. Encourage them to pay attention to their own feelings and reactions, as early recognition can prevent more severe consequences.

- **Setting Boundaries:** Guide caregivers in setting healthy boundaries to protect their time, energy, and emotional resources. Encourage them to say "no" when necessary and prioritize self-care activities. Setting boundaries can also involve creating dedicated time for self-reflection, relaxation, or engaging in activities that bring them joy and a sense of fulfillment.

- **Practicing Self-Compassion:** Teach caregivers the importance of self-compassion and self-acceptance. Encourage them to treat themselves with kindness and understanding, especially during challenging times. Help them recognize and challenge any self-critical thoughts or negative self-talk that may arise. Mindfulness and self-compassion practices can be powerful tools in fostering self-care and resilience.

- **Seeking Support:** Encourage caregivers to seek their own support systems, including individual therapy or counseling if needed. Many caregivers may benefit from processing their own emotions and experiences separately from their loved one's therapy. Support groups or peer support networks can also provide a sense of connection and validation.

- **Engaging in Enjoyable Activities:** Remind caregivers to make time for activities they find enjoyable and fulfilling. This could be engaging in hobbies, spending time in nature, connecting with friends, or pursuing personal interests. Nurturing their passions and sources of joy can replenish their emotional reserves and enhance their overall well-being.

Involving caregivers and support systems in the therapeutic process is a collaborative endeavor that strengthens the foundation for healing. By educating, supporting, and empowering caregivers, we create a network of understanding and resilience that surrounds the client. Caregivers become allies in the healing journey, equipped with the knowledge and skills to provide consistent and compassionate support. As therapists, we play a vital role in guiding and nurturing these relationships, fostering an environment that promotes growth, recovery, and the rebuilding of lives touched by trauma.

Ethical and Legal Considerations

As a therapist, one of the most crucial aspects of your work is navigating the complex landscape of ethical and legal considerations. This is especially true when treating trauma, as the sensitive nature of trauma work demands the utmost care and attention to ethical principles and legal guidelines. In this chapter, we will delve into these intricate matters, ensuring that you have a comprehensive understanding of how to ethically and legally navigate your trauma-focused CBT practice.

Confidentiality and Privacy

Confidentiality is a cornerstone of the therapeutic relationship. Creating a safe and trusting environment where clients feel secure in sharing their experiences is essential for effective trauma work. Therapists have a legal and ethical obligation to protect client confidentiality. This means that any information shared during sessions remains private and is not disclosed without the client's consent. However, it's important to be aware of exceptions to confidentiality, such as situations where there is a risk of harm to the client or others, or when required by law, such as in cases of child abuse or court-ordered disclosures. Inform your clients about these exceptions during the initial stages of therapy and have clear policies in place regarding confidentiality and privacy practices.

Mandated Reporting

Trauma therapists often work with individuals who have experienced or witnessed various forms of abuse or neglect. In such cases, mandated reporting laws come into play. As a therapist, you have a legal obligation to report suspected cases of abuse, neglect, or exploitation to the appropriate authorities. This includes situations where a client discloses abuse occurring in their family or community. Understand the mandated reporting laws in your state or country and ensure you know the designated agencies or entities to which reports should be made. While this can be a challenging aspect of the work, it is crucial for protecting vulnerable individuals and upholding legal requirements.

Informed Consent

Obtaining informed consent is a fundamental ethical principle in therapy. This means that clients must voluntarily agree to participate in treatment after being provided with comprehensive information about the nature of the therapeutic process, potential risks and benefits, fees, confidentiality policies, and their right to refuse or withdraw from treatment at any time. When working with trauma-focused CBT, it's important to explain the specific techniques and interventions that will be used, such as exposure therapy or cognitive restructuring. Ensure that clients understand the potential for emotional distress during trauma processing and that they provide consent for these therapeutic approaches. Regularly assess your client's ongoing consent throughout treatment, especially when introducing new interventions or when working with minors, as parental or guardian consent may also be necessary.

Cultural Competence

Cultural competence is an essential aspect of ethical practice in therapy. As a trauma therapist, it is your responsibility to recognize and respect the cultural backgrounds, beliefs, and values of your clients. Understand how cultural factors influence trauma responses and tailor your therapeutic approaches accordingly. This may involve incorporating cultural traditions, spiritual practices, or community support systems into the healing process. Seek ongoing training and education to enhance your cultural competence, including learning about diverse trauma responses, historical trauma, and the impact of social injustices on marginalized communities. Cultivate self-awareness by reflecting on your own cultural lens and biases, ensuring that these do not interfere with providing culturally sensitive and responsive care.

Working with Minors and Parental Involvement

When treating minors, additional ethical considerations come into play. It's important to establish a collaborative relationship with the child's parents or guardians while also respecting the client's confidentiality and autonomy. Obtain informed consent from the parents or guardians, providing them with information about the therapeutic process and your confidentiality policies. Involve the caregivers in a manner that supports the child's treatment while maintaining the child's right to privacy, especially when discussing sensitive trauma-related content. Assess the level of parental involvement needed and provide guidance to caregivers on how they can best support their child's healing journey. Remember that in certain situations, such as when a minor discloses abuse by a parent or guardian, you must follow mandated reporting procedures and ensure the safety of the child.

Record Keeping and Documentation

Accurate and thorough record keeping is both an ethical and legal requirement. Maintain detailed records of your sessions, including intake assessments, treatment plans, progress notes, and any relevant correspondence. Your documentation should reflect the client's presenting concerns, therapeutic goals, interventions used, and their progress over time. Ensure that your records are stored securely and confidentially, adhering to any applicable data protection laws and regulations. Good record-keeping not only protects you legally but also provides valuable information for treatment planning, monitoring client progress, and communicating with other professionals involved in the client's care.

Avoiding Dual Relationships

Dual relationships refer to situations where a therapist has multiple roles with a client or engages in relationships outside of the therapeutic context. These relationships can compromise the therapist's objectivity, create conflicts of interest, or lead to potential exploitation or harm. It's important to be vigilant in avoiding dual relationships, such as treating a close friend or family member, engaging in business partnerships with clients, or having social relationships that extend beyond the therapeutic frame. If a dual relationship inadvertently arises, consult with colleagues or supervisors to assess the potential risks and take steps to mitigate any negative consequences.

Maintaining Professional Boundaries

Establishing and maintaining clear professional boundaries is crucial in trauma-focused CBT. Boundaries provide a framework for the therapeutic relationship, ensuring that interactions are respectful, appropriate, and beneficial to the client's healing process. This includes being mindful of physical touch, self-disclosure, gift-giving, and the use of technology or social media. Set clear boundaries regarding session length, fees, and expectations for attendance and cancellation. While it's important to be empathetic and caring, avoid crossing boundaries that may blur the lines between therapist and friend. Clear boundaries foster a safe and effective therapeutic environment, protecting both the client and the therapist.

Consultation and Supervision

Ethical practice involves recognizing the limits of your competence and seeking consultation or supervision when needed. Consult with colleagues or seek supervision to enhance your skills, gain diverse perspectives, and ensure that you are providing the best possible care to your clients. Consultation is particularly important when working with complex trauma cases or when facing ethical dilemmas. Seek out mentors or supervisors who have expertise in trauma-focused CBT and can provide guidance on specific interventions, cultural considerations, or ethical challenges. Regular consultation not only supports your professional development but also contributes to better client outcomes.

Continuing Education and Professional Development

As a trauma therapist, it is your ethical responsibility to stay current with the latest research, therapeutic techniques, and developments in the field. Engage in ongoing continuing education and professional development activities to enhance your knowledge and skills. Seek out specialized training in trauma-focused CBT, attend conferences, webinars, or workshops, and stay connected with professional organizations that offer resources and networking opportunities. By investing in your professional growth, you ensure that your clients receive the most effective and up-to-date treatments available.

Ethical and legal considerations are integral to the practice of trauma-focused CBT. They provide a framework for delivering safe, effective, and culturally responsive care to your clients. By prioritizing confidentiality, adhering to mandated reporting laws, obtaining informed consent, and cultivating cultural competence, you create a therapeutic environment that is grounded in trust, respect, and integrity. Additionally, maintaining professional boundaries, seeking consultation, and engaging in continuous learning ensure that you remain ethically attuned and provide the highest standard of care. Ultimately, navigating these ethical and legal considerations will enable you to confidently and competently support your clients on their journey towards healing and recovery from trauma.

Conclusion
Promoting Resilience and Preventing Retraumatization

Trauma recovery is a transformative journey, and the path ahead is one of continued growth, self-discovery, and resilience building. For survivors, it's about reclaiming their sense of agency, embracing their strength, and cultivating a deep wellspring of inner resources to draw upon. This chapter aims to provide a comprehensive roadmap for ongoing healing and a bright beacon to guide survivors towards a future filled with hope, purpose, and joy.

Resilience is the remarkable capacity to adapt and bounce back from adversity, and it forms the very core of successful trauma recovery. Nurturing resilience is about fostering a mindset that embraces challenges as opportunities for growth. It involves encouraging survivors to view themselves as capable, resilient beings who possess the inner strength to navigate life's ups and downs. This mindset shift empowers them to approach their healing journey with a sense of agency and optimism.

Encourage survivors to reflect on their strengths and past successes, no matter how small they may seem. Highlight their resilience in overcoming previous challenges and emphasize how these experiences have equipped them with valuable coping skills. By recognizing and acknowledging their inherent resilience, survivors can begin to trust in their ability to handle future difficulties.

Surrounding oneself with a supportive network is a cornerstone of resilience and long-term healing. Encouraging survivors to cultivate meaningful relationships and seek out positive social connections is vital. This may include family members, close friends, support groups, or therapeutic communities. These relationships provide a sense of belonging, validation, and understanding, fostering a sense of safety and acceptance. Additionally, mentors or role models who have experienced similar traumas and successfully navigated their healing journeys can offer invaluable guidance and inspiration.

Teaching survivors effective self-care practices and healthy coping strategies is essential for resilience and preventing retraumatization. Guide them to explore a variety of self-soothing techniques, such as mindfulness meditation, deep breathing exercises, yoga, or creative outlets like journaling and art. Encourage survivors to identify activities that bring them joy and a sense of accomplishment, whether it's engaging in nature, practicing a hobby, or volunteering. These positive experiences and healthy coping mechanisms enhance emotional regulation, build resilience, and provide a buffer against stress and potential triggers.

Equipping survivors with skills to manage their emotional responses is crucial. Teach them to recognize the signs of escalating emotions and provide strategies to calm themselves down. This may include techniques such as progressive muscle relaxation, grounding exercises, or safe spaces imagery. Additionally, distress tolerance skills, such as distraction, self-soothing, and radical acceptance, can help survivors navigate intense emotions without resorting to unhealthy coping mechanisms. By improving emotional regulation, survivors can enhance their resilience and reduce the risk of retraumatization.

Challenging Negative Thought Patterns

Trauma often leaves survivors with distorted thinking patterns, such as negative self-talk, all-or-nothing thinking, or catastrophic interpretations. Encouraging survivors to challenge these unhelpful thoughts and replace them with more balanced perspectives fosters resilience. Teach them to identify cognitive distortions and practice reframing their thoughts in a more realistic and self-compassionate light. By adopting a more flexible and positive mindset, survivors can build resilience against future stressors.

Setting Boundaries and Assertive Communication

Empower survivors to set healthy boundaries and practice assertive communication. Often, trauma survivors struggle with asserting their needs and protecting themselves from potentially harmful situations. Teach them to recognize their personal limits and practice expressing their wants and boundaries clearly and respectfully. By setting boundaries, survivors can safeguard their emotional well-being and reduce the likelihood of retraumatization.

Mindfulness practices have proven benefits for trauma recovery and resilience building. Encourage survivors to incorporate mindfulness into their daily lives, focusing on the present moment without judgment. Mindfulness helps survivors become more attuned to their thoughts, emotions, and bodily sensations, allowing them to respond skillfully rather than reacting impulsively. Grounding techniques, such as the 5-4-3-2-1 coping skill or mindful walking, can anchor survivors in the here and now, enhancing their sense of stability and resilience.

Gratitude and Self-Compassion

Cultivating an attitude of gratitude can significantly enhance resilience and well-being. Encourage survivors to reflect on the positive aspects of their lives and express gratitude for even the smallest blessings. Additionally, self-compassion is a vital aspect of resilience. Teach survivors to treat themselves with kindness and understanding, recognizing that they are doing the best they can. Self-compassion involves offering oneself the same empathy and support one would extend to a dear friend.

Embracing Growth and Post-Traumatic Growth

Post-traumatic growth is the phenomenon of personal growth and transformation that can arise from the struggle with trauma. Help survivors recognize the potential for growth and encourage them to embrace the lessons learned from their trauma journey. This may include increased resilience, a deeper sense of empathy, a heightened appreciation for life, or a stronger sense of personal strength. By viewing their trauma as an opportunity for growth, survivors can find meaning and purpose in their experiences.

Preventing Retraumatization

An essential aspect of long-term healing is preventing retraumatization. This involves equipping survivors with the knowledge and skills to identify and avoid potential triggers, as well as manage their responses to triggering situations. Educate survivors about common triggers, such as specific environments, sensory stimuli, or interpersonal dynamics, and help them develop personalized strategies to navigate these triggers effectively. This may include creating safety plans, utilizing grounding techniques, or seeking support from their network.

Advocacy and Self-Advocacy

Empower survivors to become their own advocates. Encourage them to speak up for themselves, assert their needs, and seek support when necessary. Teach survivors about their rights, especially in contexts such as healthcare, education, and the legal system. By advocating for themselves, survivors can actively participate in their healing journey and ensure their voices are heard.

Continuing the Healing Journey

Healing from trauma is not a linear process, and setbacks or triggers may arise along the way. Reassure survivors that challenges and setbacks are normal and provide them with strategies to manage these obstacles effectively. Encourage survivors to maintain their therapeutic gains by continuing their self-care practices, staying connected to their support systems, and seeking ongoing therapy or support groups if needed. Emphasize that healing is an ongoing journey, and they can always return to the tools and insights gained during their trauma recovery process.

Leaving a Legacy of Hope

Finally, encourage survivors to pay it forward by sharing their stories, offering support to others, or advocating for trauma-informed practices in their communities. Leaving a legacy of hope involves recognizing the power of their own recovery and using it to inspire and uplift others. This may involve mentoring, volunteering, or simply sharing their experiences to raise awareness and break the stigma surrounding trauma.

As we bring this guide to a close, remember that healing is an art, and resilience is the palette with which survivors paint their future. It is my sincere hope that the insights and tools shared in these pages will accompany you on your continued journey towards healing and empowering others. May you carry the light of resilience, illuminating the path for yourself and those you touch, fostering a world where trauma is understood, addressed, and transformed into a catalyst for growth and positive change.

NOTE

NOTE

NOTE

NOTE

NOTE

NOTE

www.ingramcontent.com/pod-product-compliance
Lightning Source LLC
Chambersburg PA
CBHW071943210526
45479CB00002B/791